HOW TO HAVE A PHONE SEX

:A beginners guide to having hot and fun intimacy online

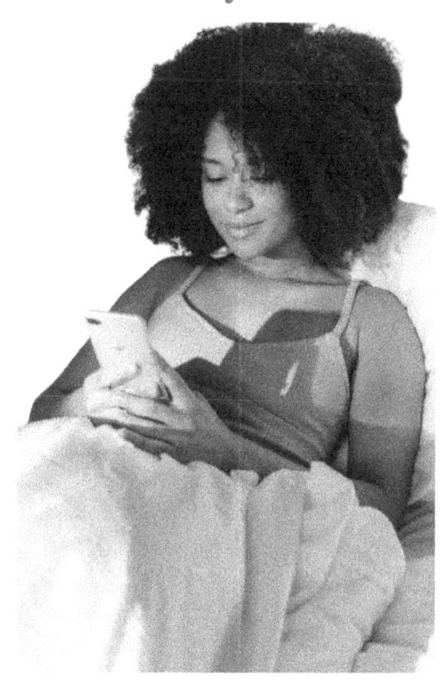

Linda K. Montana

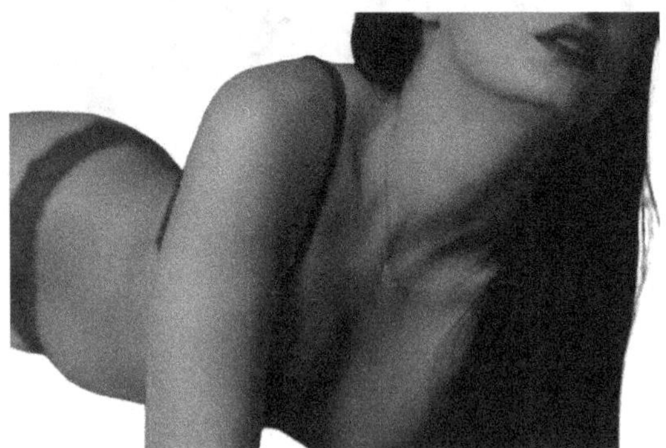

TABLE OF CONTENT

Introduction

phone sex is an extraordinary method for enlivening your sexual coexistence, whether you're doing it in light of the fact that your partner is far away, in light of the fact that you're not prepared to have different sorts of sex yet, on the grounds that you simply need to take a stab at something new, or for some other explanation!

To have extraordinary phone sex, you want to set free, quit being hesitant, and be prepared to get turned on, regardless of how senseless you might feel right away.

Chapter 1 : Getting ready

Stage 1: How to Set up a phone date.

While the facts really confirm that, likewise with some other sort of sex, phone sex can "simply occur", the meeting is bound to work out positively assuming you've prepared, particularly assuming that it's your most memorable time doing it together.

Pick when you're both alone and allowed to set your restraints free. Your arrangement won't work in the event that you're moving around in bed, feeling hot and weighty, while your partner is shuddering in the downpour outside the library.

Assuming your partneris new to phone sex or feeling uncertain, think about sending them this article, or perusing it together.

Remember that you can constantly talk about what you might want to do during phone sex before you start.

Stage 2 : How to Set Free and get in that Frame of mind.

It will be hard for you to have fun assuming you feel tense or senseless, so before you call, do anything you want to do to get yourself familiar and feeling hot.

Set free: Lie in bed for some time, peruse the web, have a glass of wine, run on the spot, do a senseless routine before the mirror,

anything that will permit you to set the pressure free from your body.

Get in that frame of mind: Setting up a provocative environment can assist with placing you in the right outlook, so consider doing anything that you'd do to plan for some other sort of sex.

Here are a few thoughts:

Clean up your room and make the bed

Faint the lights, maybe set up certain candles

Play delicate music

Have a shower or shower (and a shave, if that you like)

Consider pretending to brighten up the call (both of you think plunging, and so on.)

Put on (or take off!) your number one, hottest garments, and clothing

Set out some sex toys

Turn yourself on by tenderly stroking your body, or pondering your sweetheart, or envisioning sexual experiences you've had or might want to have... in any case, don't allow yourself to get excessively turned on presently - - that is the very thing the call is for!

Chapter 2: Starting a phone Sex

1. How to Start the call.

When you have your partner on the phone, take things at a speed you're both OK with. There's no "right" method for having phone sex.

In the event that it assists you with unwinding, put in almost no time visiting before you get everything rolling... simply don't allow yourselves to get diverted from your attractive objective.

A low, delicate manner of speaking or weighty breathing can assist with setting the state of mind, however don't drive it in the event that doing so is unnatural for you: talking and breathing easily in your ordinary manner of speaking will be hotter than an ungracefully constrained endeavor at sounding hot.

2. How to start with a hot topic

Present a relaxed subject that will segue pleasantly into provocative talk. Getting everything rolling is potentially the hardest part, particularly in the event that it's your most memorable time! Pick a point that is simple for you to raise, however which can possibly twist into a steamier area.

Examples:

The amount you miss them, or wish they were with you

What you might want to do assuming that they were with you

What you're wearing and the way that you thoroughly search in it

What you're doing

How you're feeling

Request that your partner portray any of the above to you

3. How to Grow more into hot talk

When you have the ball rolling and you're feeling great, take a stab at getting bolder with your depictions, or raise new, hotter points. A decent methodology is to portray or request that your partner depict, the accompanying three things:

What you're doing: Depict what you look like and the manner in which you're contacting yourself. Be as bashful or as ignoble as you like!

Request "guidance" for instance, "would it be a good idea for me to begin playing with my clothing?"

Let them know what you'd like them to do in the event that they're willing.

Try not to feel awful if you're not happy with contacting yourself - you can in any case tell them that you're appreciating, essentially paying attention to them.

What you're envisioning: This could be, for instance, how you might want to do your accomplice, a second from extraordinary sex you two have had previously, or a psychological picture of what they're depicting to you.

You should begin slow: start with tame portrayals like "first, I'd stroke your hair" or "I truly like the manner in which your chest thoroughly searches in a Shirt", prior to continuing on toward steamier things like "then I'd kiss your neck" or "recollect when you did that thing to me in the shower?"

As usual, how unequivocal you get, and how rapidly, is completely dependent upon you.

How you're feeling: Portray the physical and profound sentiments you're encountering because of what you're doing or potentially what they're talking about.

Groaning is an extraordinary method for conveying how great you're feeling.

In any case, there's a compelling reason you need to do this in the event that you're not happy with it. You can begin with simply allowing your breath to go from the get go, to assist with bringing out little groans into stronger groans.

Tell them when they've depicted or accomplished something you truly appreciated. In like manner, make it a point to let them know when you loathe something - it'll permit you two to continue on toward something different that you'll both view as charming.

Educate me regarding your sexual dreams: Portraying your sexual dreams permits you to illustrate their dreams.

Allow your partner to stand up clearly about their dreams and you can do likewise.

4. How to Masturbate and climax during phone sex

Common masturbation and climax are great increments to phone sex, yet they're not a necessity using any and all means.

Try not to feel awful if that your partner doesn't go along with you in stroking off. To stroke off alone, ask them before you start assuming they'd be keen on going along with you. Similarly, don't get restless in the event that they begin jerking off and you would rather not - - you're not committed to go along with them. Simply appreciate paying attention to them and delight themselves.

Just relax in the event that either of you neglect to arrive at the climax. Consider it the good to beat all, as opposed to the objective of the activity.

Assuming you arrive at climax before your partneris prepared to stop, don't go calm! Keep conversing with them, depicting what you're feeling and envisioning.

5. How to Get Done with Having Phone sex.

The place where you choose to stop depends on you. There's a compelling reason to sit tight for climax or, without a doubt, to stop since you've both come.

There's no standard regarding how rapidly you ought to end the call in the wake of wrapping up.

Certain individuals favor finishing the call when their breathing has returned to ordinary, though others like to remain available and visit.

Tell your partner the amount you had a ball before you end the call.

Chapter 3:Questions

How can I arouse a young lady via phone?

Don't hesitate for even a moment to utilize your creative mind! Dial up the tomfoolery by asking something like: " Assuming nothing was forbidden and it could be incredible regardless, how might you need to manage me physically that we haven't previously?"

Is there any damage in having phone sex consistently?

Not actually, no. Since it's via phone, there is clearly no possibility of pregnancy or sexually transmitted diseases. Simply ensure you (and your accomplice) are not feeling constrained to do anything you/they would rather not do.

How could couples do this in any case?

For what reason might they at any point do this, in actuality?
Perhaps if the spouse/sweetheart or wife/sweetheart is away somewhere and the individual they are dating believes they should do it with them yet can't.

For this situation, phone sex could feel like they are being personal from a remote place. There are numerous potential motivations behind why however, it's private and between the consenting accomplices.

Chapter 4: Bonus

19 Hints to Assist You With having the Most sultry and hot phone Sex of Your Life

Hot phone sex isn't an ironic expression — it's valid!

"Somebody's voice and groans can genuinely stimulate,"

Also, while your accomplice's hand/tongue/pieces may not be Accessible For Use, your own hands and joy items are not too far off if you have them and need to utilize them!

Phone sex can be a hot method for having intercourse with somebody, similar to a Kindling match or previous school colleague, without destroying the dream.

1. Request for consent from your partner

What's more, not simply once.

Do a temperature check
"At the point when you're in a casual setting, put the thought out there and perceive how they answer it,"

Far to bring it up face to face:

"It's obvious I won't see you for a couple of days after this. I was figuring it very well may be amusing to attempt phone sex before we see each other once more."

"My friend was simply letting me know that she and her partner have phone sex. It's not something I've had previously, however I may be keen on attempting assuming you are. Do you have any considerations about phone sex?"

Assuming their response is "perhaps" and they appear to be apprehensive or reluctant, you could get some information about having phone sex that they're uncertain of.

In the event that it's the absence of visuals, you could attempt a video call all things being equal. if it's having the option to talk provocatively, you could begin by sexting.

if that you're not truly with the other individual, you could bring it up with:

"Is phone sex something you are willing to try out together?"

"At any point are you keen on jolting off while I'm on the other line? I think paying attention to one another getting off could be truly hot."

Furthermore, if that you're asking a sexting mate or Kindling match you haven't yet met?

Is this a totally freakish inquiry, or have your discussions previously been expressly sexual?

if that you have a virtual indulgence, you could send a message that says:
"I've adored speaking profanely with you over text. Hearing your voice express these things would seriously turn me on. Might I at any point take you on a phone sex date?"

"Are you willing to move these filthy discussions from message to phone? I'd very much want to hear you groan."

Ask assent before a particular phone sex meeting, as well

Before you murmur to your accomplice, "I need to lick and suck you until you're pretty much as dry as the Sahara Desert," you really want to ensure that they're down to filthy talk right this exact second.

That will save you from the ponderousness of laying everything out there when your partner is generally distracted — like assuming they're working or with their folks.

In addition, there's no rollover impact with assent. " You want to inquire as to whether your partner needs to have phone sex each and every time,"

You don't have to plan it weeks ahead of time — however a week after week phone sex date isn't an ill-conceived notion for you LDR people.

A "Hey! What are you doing this evening? Might I at any point entice you to a phone sex date?" or on the other hand "I've been contemplating the manner in which you sound when you come throughout the morning. Do you possess energy for a filthy talk date in the not so distant future?" will guarantee you're both in total agreement.

2. Connect about language

Never is language so significant than when you're nose-somewhere down in your accomplice's overlap and... you get the point.

Get some information about body inclination words
Fam, before you have any sort of hot relations with somebody — face to face, video, text, or call — you ought to figure out what things and descriptors they like for their pieces and sways.

"Figure out what words cause them to feel hot and feel better,"

The most straightforward method for doing that? Share what words you like. For instance:

"I love it when you call my pussy a pussy or vagina, yet I have a bad relationship with c*nt. What words feel best to you?"
"I truly like when you wax graceful about how solid and strong my back is the point at which I give you head, yet I could do without the word 'cumbersome.' Are there any words you either truly like or could do without?"
Another choice: Seek your partner for language prompts
Except if you're additionally a sex essayist or sex instructor, odds are good that you've never asked somebody

(or been asked yourself) what body part words they like.

So if your partner offers you a non-response to the abovementioned, there's another option: Stand by listening to how they reference their own bodies.

Odds are eventually your partner will tell you they're [verbing] their [noun].

Monitor what those action words and things are, and use them while depicting you're doing to their [noun].

3. Find out more about the language of lovemaking

On account of the wretched sex schooling in the US, the majority of our sexicon doesn't go past "vagina," "bosoms," "condom," and "sex."

"If you're not used to discussing sex or your body in nonmedical ways, phone sex will be more diligently,"

It is suggested extending your verbiage with the assistance of the beneath:
A sexting robot
That's right! This exists. Sex and relationship application Juicebox delivered a component called Slutbox which permits you to improve your messy talk abilities — or simply get some horny cherishing while you're feeling forlorn.

4. Understand erotica

What could be a superior method for increasing your messy word reference passages than with some page pornography? Either select more limited, online stories from locales like Sugar Butch Narratives and Aurore, or read an all out suggestive book.

Here are some A+ erotica books that you can try reading

"Fifty Shades of Dark":

"The Chief" by Abigail Barnette

"The Club" by A.L. Streams

"No Restrictions" by Lori Cultivate

"Journal of a Compliant" by Sophie Morgan

"The Programmer Series" by Meredith Wild

"To Italy With Adoration" by Fiona Zedde

5. Pay attention to sound erotica

Like understanding erotica, paying attention to it opens you to action words, things, and descriptors you can acquire for your own sensual scenes.

In addition, it'll get you used to hearing the very hot expressions.

Some famous sound erotica locales and applications:

Dipsea

Quinn

Girl on the Net

Bawdy Storytelling

Put on porn... yet don't watch it

Simply tune in. CrashPadSeries is a particularly decent (paid) pornography site for learning ascent based, delight centered phrases.

6. Set everything up

Regardless of whether you never plan to acquaint video with your sex sesh, you really want to restrict interruptions,

Assuming you're focusing on the feline or browsing the email warning that just sprung up on your phone, your partner will detect that you're distracted.

Make the accompanying strides for set up:

Flip your phone to Don't Upset mode, and mood killer any remaining innovation.

Clean your room.

Set the space to an agreeable temp.

Put your pleasure props in a simple to-arrive place.

Play tunes, staying away from locales that play advertisements.

Light candles and faint the lights.

7. Getting everything rolling

Your room is perfect, you have your corrupted word reference in your back pocket (except if you've proactively dropped trou) and approval from your partner to phone bone. What's the deal? There are a couple of choices.

8. Mutually masturbate

Shed your skivvies and arrive at between your legs. Or on the other hand, get your numero uno buzzy pal.

Then, with your phone in one hand and your garbage or toy in the other, have at it!

"phone sex doesn't need to be intricate,".

" Paying attention to the smallest sounds and groans of the other person groaning can be exciting absent a lot of other talking."

9. Explain everything you are doing

From taking your shirt off to sliding a finger inside one of your openings, "Telling your partner bit by bit through the thing you're doing and the way that you're touching yourself can be hot."

Her tip: Go sluggish. As opposed to promptly connecting your Enchanted Wand and making wizardry, begin by letting your partner know where you are, what you're wearing, and the way that horny you've been day in and day out.

Then, get definite. Extremely point by point. Summon however many faculties as you can with your portrayals, it proposes. For example, "The lubricant feels cool against my clit."

10. Remember a past frolic

"The words 'recall when' are an extraordinary method for beginning provocative talking,". " Then, you and your partner can cooperate to recap the experience."

Once more, go sluggish. Try not to say, for instance, "Recollect when we beat on the soccer field for like 3 hours, that was entertaining."

It doesn't give your partner much to answer.

All things being equal, carry your partner into the narrating experience.

"Do you remember that time on the soccer field? The night it was cold, and we were the only ones around and you provided me with that look of yours prior to maneuvering me onto the grass?"

The thing that matters is unobtrusive yet powerful!

"Questions are an incredible instrument for making all the difference for the discussion,"

Recapping works best as a gathering exercise with somebody you've previously had IRL sex with.

In the event that your partner has a cuckolding dream, and they impart that they need you to, you can educate them regarding an involvement in another person.

11. Explore the world of fantasy

"phone sex can be a great method for discussing things you and your partner are willing to do together, all things considered,". For example, "Assuming both of you have discussed having a trio previously, talk through what that would resemble."

Phone sex can likewise be a tomfoolery space to fantasize about things you never really need to occur.

For instance, perhaps you track down a two fold entrance excruciating face to face, however I think the dream of completion is hot.

Warning: " Make sure your partner comprehends the distinction between a dream you most certainly need to attempt, should attempt under the right conditions, and most certainly don't have any desire to attempt."

12. Seek clarification on pressing issues

It is suggested beginning here assuming that you've as of late begun engaging in sexual relations with this individual, or never have.

"It's an effective method for getting a feeling of their opinion on sex,".

What to inquire:

"Can you share your thought process regarding the last time you masturbated?"

"What was the most amazing sexual experience you've had at any point?"
"What are you wearing?"
Keep up the moment(come)
These tips can assist you with keeping G-O-ing once you begin.

13. Try not to rush it

"Similarly as sex is typically best when slow, so is phone sex,".

Hold your rhythm and use suspension and expectation to spice things up."

14. Laugh!

As opposed to being an indication that things are going south, "giggling is a sign you're OK with one another and living it up,".

"Sex shouldn't be so serious. Embrace the delight."

15. Be you

Except if you and your partner are explicitly pretending a dream that expects you to modify the pitch of your voice or claim to be a ruler from a distant land, there's a compelling reason you need to do that.

if that there's a respite in the convo "A break in a discussion can occur if a partner is feeling hesitant, so get some information about, or what they're feeling at that moment,".

Indeed "Is this actually feeling better to you?" works.

You could likewise utilize this opportunity to let your partner know how you would contact them if you were there.

"Let's say you're feeling the vibes and you get the feeling that your partner is feeling compliant, you can let them know how to touch themselves, or what toy to utilize,".

16. Another choice: Begin groaning!

"Simply masturbate and allow your partner to hear you,". " It'll be a good time for both of you."

Imagine a scenario where something isn't working.

Say so. A few lines to help divert the convo:

"This evening I'd like it if you'd XYZ."

"Will you be available to XYZ in all things considered?"

"I don't need that at this moment. In any case, perhaps after you XYZ."

Assuming they offered something that has totally removed you from it, tell them. For instance:

"Hey, Please accept my apologies for doing this, however that one line removed me from the scenario.

"I'm struggling with staying alone at the time, would you like to discuss something somewhat less hot or hang up?"

"I have a past filled with bad memories and what you only said brought that up for me, so I really want to eliminate myself from this discussion. I want to believe that you accept."

17. Include video

It's quite simple to go from voice to voice in addition to video. Cheers to innovation!

However long you and your partner are similarly into it, go ahead and signal up video and let your eyes devour the hot human you've been envisioning the entire evening.

18. The main concern if is not going as plan

Phone bonding has as much joy potential as some other sex.

"It could feel hawkward from the start, yet you may be surprised the way that

hot and fearless you feel behind a phone screen,"
" Embrace it!"

If that isn't working for you, recall that you can likewise stop it!

5 Last Ways to keep phone Sex Scorching

If you've perused this far, you'll have an incredible handle on how to have extraordinary phone sex with your man. These last four hints are good to beat all and will take you from a phone sex diva to a phone sex genius.

1. Be sure, to schedule It Or Not - In the event that you and your man are caught up with, booking phone dates seems OK. This is particularly evident if you have any desire to find an opportunity to prepare and in that frame of mind. Notwithstanding, occasionally, improvised phone sex can be hot as well. My recommendation is to attempt both and center around what turns out best for both of you.

2. Slow, Enticing and Hot Voice - In Section 2 of the Grimy Talking Guide, I discuss how speaking profanely is for the most part about your voice tone, the speed you talk at, and the specific situation. I examine how the genuine grimy talking phrases you use aren't close to as significant as HOW you say them.

This is critical while having phone sex with your man. It will be multiple times more powerful and provocative when you talk gradually and enticingly.

Telling wisecracks or talking super quick isn't a turn on when you are attempting to have phone sex with your man. It ruins the state of mind.

Notwithstanding, you shouldn't attempt to utilize a phony voice since it very well may occupy.

Try not to zero in such a great amount on the particulars. Accepting at least for now that you're getting everything done as needs be, your sentences might be cut off by groans and moans. What's more, the words aren't really significant when you're short of breath.

3. You're Not Working In A Call Place - What I mean by this is that you should be excited about phone sex. At the point when you get a call from a call community, the voice on the other line is normally exhausting, uninterested, apathetic, and Counterfeit. This is on the grounds that the individual calling you couldn't care less, AND they are simply pursuing a content. This sort of mentality Obliterates phone sex.

You really want to zero in on ensuring you are excited and truly appreciate paying attention to him. In the event that you are simply pursuing a content, it won't sound veritable AND you won't have the option to get criticism from your man.

A couple of arranged lines can help (and the Messy Talking Guide has a lot of models), however a whole content beginning to end that you arranged before is unavoidably going to sound phony. It additionally makes it harder to make do.

Picking a situation is a greatly improved method for moving toward phone sex. It provides you with a harsh thought of what to say during phone sex and permits you the adaptability to take it any place you believe it should go.

Make an effort not to zero in such a great amount on recalling phone sex phrases. All things being equal, simply take the path of least resistance.

That implies you or your man could offer something like
You would do that way. You're so grimy.
And keeping in mind that you do X, I'd do Y...

4. It's alright To Be awkward! - While you're figuring out how to have great phone sex with your man, you'll have to escape your usual range of familiarity and at times this can get a bit abnormal. You can definitely relax; this is simply an aspect of the interaction.

This additionally implies it very well may be OK to snicker. All things considered, now and again somebody says or accomplishes something entertaining, in any event, while you're engaging in sexual relations face to face, and you should have the option to make fun of yourself. At any rate, the main thing isn't to allow it to remove you from your headspace and continue onward.

If that you let a tad of cumbersomeness keep you from proceeding, you will pass up loads of fun in the long haul. So my recommendation is simply to proceed. In time, the cumbersomeness will pass and be supplanted by hot, hot phone sex.

5. Take on a steady speed - Regardless of what you say explicitly, it's normally savvy to begin slow.

You could groan delicately, tease, or act shy from the beginning. You would rather not get very unequivocal without skipping a beat. Moving toward that makes sexual pressure that makes phone sex considerably more agreeable!

Essentially, you should begin exercises gradually. Think about it like foreplay except if, obviously, you need to attempt a quick in and out via phone!

Be that as it may, you don't need to get very expressive in the event that you would rather not. Frequently it's simpler to groan than to talk or offer something truly filthy. Obviously, your man will likely adore it assuming you do!

At the point when It's Not Working

At last, we want to discuss what to do when things end up.. not all that attractive. Perhaps the bearing of the situation isn't doing it for you, or your man has utilized a word or expression that switches you off. It's not completely like being face to face. In circumstances such as these, you could need to offer something, for example,

I'd appreciate it if we discussed X all things being equal. Could that be alright?

Apologies, I don't cherish that word. Could you at any point call it Y?

What's more, in some cases phone sex simply doesn't work for you, so you could need to tap out. All things considered, evaluate any of the accompanying.

Please accept my apologies, however my head simply isn't in the game. Might we at any point attempt this some other time?

I would rather not say it, however this isn't working for me today. Might I at any point assist you with wrapping up?

You can continuously attempt once more at a later time or on the other hand, in the event that you conclude sex on the phone isn't for you, have a go at something different.

Certain individuals favor FaceTime or Skype for their advanced sex. You could adhere to sexting or even handwrite a hot letter.

Maybe you watch pornography simultaneously as your partner, however without the sound part. It's perfect to take a stab at a novel, new thing, yet you never need to do something you would rather not.

The last comment about having phone sex with your man is that you are not limited to just utilizing your phone. Skype, FaceTime, Viber, Zoom Google Meet, and the wide range of various voice calling and VOIP applications out there make for amazing other options.

You can likewise consolidate pictures. Your voice ought to be the superstar, however you can send a couple of pictures, maybe as you strip down or even something somewhat more scandalous to support your man. Figure out how to take a hot selfie.

In the period of rapid video, you can be on camera the entire time. Attempt FaceTime sex or utilizing whatever application you like.

There's no phone sex procedure that you totally should attempt. Everything no doubt revolves around trial and error, finding what you like, and investigating with your accomplice.

Question

My man is imprisoned at the present moment and will be for the following year. He gets a kick out of the chance to have phone sex yet it's not especially something that I'm accustomed to doing and in some cases it's somewhat abnormal. In some cases I'll try and simply go about as though I'm doing the things he is requesting that I do different times I do them. How might I turn out to be more agreeable for my man?

Reply

1 method is to figure out what you Truly do like at the chance to do with regards to phone sex and doing that.

Question

I felt somewhat anxious having facetime phone sex... . I got the womanizer team vibrator. It is costly. Yet, OMFG. You won't feel humiliated any longer you will simply be shouting and cumming and thinking how much fun it is...

Reply

Additionally, assuming that it is legitimate where you are, doing weed during it is considerably more tomfoolery !

Question

I generally have phone sex with my sweetheart. We have a remote relationship with him and when we are doing it on the phone he's the person who speaks profanely. I'm simply there saying daddy he groans yet I have no clue assuming that they are genuine groans. What's more, I generally get modest while making it happen. In some cases I keep silent and not groan, different times I simply leave him and hang up. yikes and at whatever point he maintains that should do it im consistently bustling like guardians are home or I would rather not be clear he generally lashes out and stuff yet I don't have the foggiest idea how to tell him i'm consistently occupied.

Question

I'm in LDR. We have video sex yet it has flamed out in light of the fact that I continually feel abnormal. I'm terrible at talking grimy in light of the fact that I never need to sound ludicrous. I watch out not to start again on the grounds that I'm abnormal. It's been 11 years for me really having actual sex with anybody and to express I'm withdrawn from my sexuality is putting it mildly along these lines and presently my sexual coexistence in my LDR has dwindled along these lines. He says he maintains that I should begin starting so he has halted. I don't have the foggiest idea how to take the main action. Assist me with satisfying

Reply

Sorry to learn that. The least demanding method for having phone sex is to simply jerk off and keep the phone near your mouth with the goal that your man can hear your breath/groaning.

Experience

I had interesting phone sex interestingly recently. He's hitched so he messaged me on his break asking me when he could call. I said "whenever" and he inquired "presently?" I said it's okay and he called and asked where I was. " In My room." " What are you wearing?" " Nothing, where are you?" " In my vehicle. My rooster is getting hard contemplating you".

He was letting me know how he was removing it from his jeans so I began depicting how I was running my tongue up his rooster to his balls and all the other things. I was energized and began jerking off and we conversed with one another through it. OMG!!! I spurted again and again and drenched my pad! It was fucking perfect! My most memorable time was exceptionally fruitful. Can hardly hold on to experience it again!

Question

Recently my beau was becoming horny and began letting me know that he needed to embrace me, kiss me and so on and so on . I was feeling excessively sexual however I was timid about whether he would pass judgment on me for this if I could converse with him and I just said we should stop and I turned off the phone.

Am I thinking right or would it be advisable for me to partake in this cozy inclination with my sweetheart without a second thought.

Kindly response me

Reply

At last, you should pursue that choice yourself. Nothing bad can really be said about 2 consenting grown-ups partaking in one another physically.

Question

I have been in a phone sex relationship with a person for 3.5 years? We have never done video calls too, just talked and have been to each dream of it. Are we ordinary ?

Reply

In the event that you are both cheerful and not violating any regulations, then it seems natural to me.